Vita-Guard Keto Foods

The Newest Trend in Weight Loss

Raymond E. Smith

Published by

Sanway International 91 E. Main Street Inman, SC 29349

Email: vitaguard1912@gmail.com

Dedication to

My friend Freida Edgens

Introduction

What "keto" means

The "keto" in a ketogenic diet comes from the fact that it allows the body to produce small fuel molecules called "ketones".

This is an alternative fuel source for the body, used when blood sugar (glucose) is in short supply.

Ketones are produced if you eat very few carbs (that are quickly broken down into blood sugar) and only moderate amounts of protein (excess protein can also be converted to blood sugar).

The liver produces ketones from fat. These ketones then serve as a fuel source throughout the body, especially for the energy every day, and it can't run on fat directly. It can only run on glucose… or ketones.

On a ketogenic diet, your entire body switches its fuel supply to run mostly on fat, burning fat 24-7. When insulin levels become very low, fat burning can increase dramatically. It becomes easier to access your fat stores to burn them off.

The "keto" in a ketogenic diet comes from the fact that it allows the body to produce small fuel molecules called "ketones".

Best Keto Foods for Weight Loss

The Keto method of weight loss is probably the biggest news about weight loss in many, many years. Every investor on the panel of the TV show, Shark Tank invested millions of dollars each to turn the product into a multi-million dollars company.

This book is to show a few foods one should eat to get results from the Vita-Guard Weight Loss plan.

Going to the grocery store is a hard enough task without the added work of shopping for specific items because you're adhering to a very particular food plan. If you're following a Vita-Guard Keto Diet the aisles in search of items that the high-fat, low-carb lifestyle allows can be even trickier.

So what are some of the things you want to make sure find their way into your cart?

Don't expect to stock up on all these items immediately, but the sooner you can the better off you will be.

Why did the keto diet become so trendy for weight loss?

Believe it or not, the keto diet was originally designed to help people who suffer from seizure disorders—not to help people lose weight, says New York-based R.D. Jessica Cording. That's because both ketones and another chemical produced by the diet, called decanoic acid, may help minimize seizures.

But people who started following the keto diet noticed weight loss for a few reasons: When you eat carbs, your body retains fluid in order to store carbs for energy (you know, in case it needs it). But when you're not having much in the carb department, you lose this water weight, says Warren. Also, it's easy to go overboard on carbohydrates—but if you're loading up on fat, it may help curb cravings since it keeps you satisfied.

Things you need to do:

1. Read the Vita-Guard Weight Loss book as quickly as you can. Everything in the book is not about weight loss. It show you that anything can be accomplished when you have prepared your mind to do it.

2. Order the Vita-Guard Weight Loss Formula and take according to directions.

3. Stick to the food list to get the best results.

4. Drink 8 glasses of water each day.

Avocados

"Nearly all the calories in an avocado come from fat, and one whole fruit has less than 3 grams of digestible carbohydrate — traits that make it a perfect keto food right off the bat," Plus, avocados are high in fiber, referring to "net carbohydrates" which is found by subtracting your total fiber intake from your total grams of carbohydrates.

Other popular keto-approved veggies you'll want to consider: kale, fennel celery, cucumber, cauliflower, broccoli, bell peppers, and zucchini.

Canned Sardines

High in omega-3 fatty acids and a high-quality source of protein, canned sardines are a tasty keto staple. Plus, they also often come canned in olive oil, providing a healthy dose of fat. She adds: "And they're ready -to-eat — a claim that few keto foods can make!" Toss a couple on top of that spicy salad you're working on, and voila: that's a keto-friendly meal, which is missing in a lot of keto diets, a lack that can lead to constipation. They also kick up the potassium, and they're kind of perfect.

Bonus? That dose of fiber helps you feel full, longer. Try adding avocado slices to your salad or just eating on its own. Try cutting one open and sprinkling with sea salt before digging in.

Spinach

Unlike some other high-protein, low-carb diets, large quantities of leafy greens are not fair game on a ketogenic diet Instead, they get counted along with any other carbohydrates that you incorporate. But you'll want to include them on your keto shopping list because the plan allows for 20-30 grams of carbs per day or less to stay in ketosis, and greens can fulfill that quota.

"Each has less than half a gram of net carbs per cup, so a 4-cup salad has less than 2 grams of net carbs,"

Salmon

Then again, if the mere idea of sardines makes you cringe, salmon is a palatable alternative. "Fatty fish are an important contribution to any diet because of their uniquely high omega-3 fat content. This is especially important to a ketogenic dieter who gets most of their calories from fat. By adding that other fatty fish options include mackerel and tuna.

Olive oil

It's true that coconut oil is the "darling of the keto diet" as a result of its high MCT (medium-chain triglycerides) content, but olive oil shouldn't be overlooked. Almost 75 percent of the fats in olive oil (and olives) are the monounsaturated kind associated with good heart health.

The great thing about olive oil is there are so many varieties of olives used to make it, so the flavor profiles of different oils vary widely," There are herbaceous olive oils, ones with earthy flavors, and even some that are spicy. "A ketogenic diet can tend to lack flavor variety, so these oils can be used to spice up a dinner plate and add fat at the same time."

Flax Crackers

If you are going keto, then you can expect to miss one thing during your meals — crunch.

"If you think about it, most crunchy foods are high in carbohydrate (e.g. tortilla chips and crackers), and most fatty foods have a smooth, silky texture (e.g. avocado, mayonnaise). If you're seeking crunch, find yourself some flax crackers. These crackers have 1 to 2 grams of net carb per serving and are made entirely from flax seeds."

Well-marbled Steak

When shopping for meat look for well-marbled cuts, like a ribeye or a NY strip. And the reason for this one is pretty simple: "When you're eating a ketogenic diet, it's often hard to get enough fat and avoid over-eating protein." That way, you'll be able to eat a smaller portion of meat because the fat throughout the cut will contribute to your feeling of fullness.

Other popular protein sources on the keto diet include lamb, chicken, venison, turkey, tuna, cod and, you guessed it — bacon.

Almond Butter

"If you're already on a ketogenic diet, then you know it can require a good deal of cooking since there are so few keto-compliant prepared foods,"

Almond butter

A keto lifestyle staple that "rescues many a keto dieter from the work of meal prep.

"Not that I am recommending almond butter in lieu of a real meal, but it will do just fine as a snack in a pinch. Try putting it on celery sticks if you want the crunch. Two tablespoons (one serving) provide 18 grams of fat, 7 grams of protein and only 3 grams of net carbs."

Eggs

A lot of people, especially those on low-carb and keto diets, do 5 Days of Egg Fast to break their weight loss stall. Surprisingly, it works for a majority of them if we are to believe what they report on social networks and forums.

Try eating eggs and a meat for breakfast, nothing else. Not only will it help with your weight loss it will lower Blood sugar.

In theory, by sticking to this keto eggs formula, you'll be consuming a healthy balance of macronutrients that are extremely low carb and high fat and which contain only a moderate amount of protein. Sounds familiar? It should. Because that is necessarily what the low-carb lifestyle is. So why does the egg fast work to lose weight? And how can you survive without vegetables?

The answer to the first question is, as we mentioned, not clear. All we have to go on at this point is a mountain of anecdotal evidence that it does work since there's a lack of scientific evidence to back up those numerous assertions. As for the second question, the answer, of course, is that you can't. Or at least you can't expect to maintain anything like reasonable health if you never eat vegetables. That is one reason the egg fast lasts less than a week. Longer than that and you might be playing some serious games with your health.

One of the lesser-known aspects of being on the lowcarb lifestyle for any length of time is that, in a small number of cases, weight loss can slow to a crawl or even stall completely. In instances when this happens most people react in one of two ways: either they come to the conclusion that the keto lifestyle doesn't work after all or they look for some method of clearing the weight loss logjam to get back on the path to a leaner, healthier, more efficient body. One of the best ways to do the latter is what's called the "egg fast" or the "egg diet for keto."

During this period, you eat a minimum of 5 or 6 eggs every day along with a tablespoon of fat for each of the eggs you eat. Also, the amount of cheese you consume in ounces based on your meal plans should be less than the number of eggs you eat on any given day. So, say you eat 7 eggs one day -- that means you should not consume more than 7 ounces of full-fat cheese. If the next day you eat 5 eggs then you shouldn't eat more than 5 ounces of cheese, and so on.

One of the lesser-known aspects of being on the low carb lifestyle for any length of time is that, in a small number of cases, weight loss can slow to a crawl or even stall completely. In instances when this happens most people react in one of two ways: either they come to the conclusion that the keto lifestyle doesn't work after all or they look for some method of clearing the weight loss logjam to get back on the path to a leaner, healthier, more efficient body. One of the best ways to do the latter is what's called the "egg fast" or the "egg diet for keto."

During this period, you eat a minimum of 5 or 6 eggs every day along with a tablespoon of fat for each of the eggs you eat. Also, the amount of cheese you consume in ounces based on your meal plans should be less than the number of eggs you eat on any given day. So, say you eat 7 eggs one day -- that means you should not consume more than 7 ounces of full-fat cheese. If the next day you eat 5 eggs then you shouldn't eat more than 5 ounces of cheese, and so on.

This transport nutrients in and out of cells. And when you stop eating processed grains and sugar, you often get much less sodium. So when you go keto, just be sure that you're eating salt or sodium-rich foods. If not, you will often experience fatigue.

Eat Enough. Normally, this probably isn't a problem for you. But when you go on a keto diet, it's actually, easy to start under-eating. So every few days, just check in that you've been eating enough food.

Eat Enough Fat. Remember, most of your calories (70-85%) should be from fat. So don't skimp on the fat. If you're feeling hungry or like you need to snack, then eating more fat at meals will normally solve that problem. In general, choose the fattier cuts of meat.

So, what you need to do is learn which foods

you can and cannot consume, and also when you buy food, always make sure to check the label on the back and look for any hidden Keto-unfriendly ingredients.

Sugar Substitutes

Using sugar substitutes and sweeteners are kind of related to the previous hidden carbs section.

As it is the case for food and drinks, the main thing we are looking for in a sweetener is that, when consumed, it needs to have minimal to no impact on blood glucose and insulin levels. And there are a lot of them that don't make the cut, so to speak, including some zerocalorie sweeteners.. Stevia, Monk Fruit, Allulose, and erythritol are among the few which are safe to consume on Keto. There are also a handful of other new sweeteners on the market, but before you use one, you need to do proper research on it and make sure it meets the requirements.

And to note, it's perfectly ok to use sweeteners in moderation to satisfy your sweet tooth, but consuming them all day long is not a real solution. When you manage to get "fat adapted" and reach ketosis, your hunger and cravings for carbs will go way down any-way.

Not eating enough fat

Other than consuming too many carbs, not eat-ing enough fat can also throw you off balance and cre-ate issues. Dietary fat is essential on Keto primarily for two reasons:

Both dietary and your own fat are now your body's primary energy fuel, especially when fully "fat adapted." If you are regularly not consuming as much fat as your body needs, you will start experiencing symptoms like very low energy, fatigue, hunger, crav-ings, headaches, etc.

Healthy fats are needed to build, repair and maintain vital membranes for all cells in the body.

Just note that it is not just about quantity, but also about the quality of fats you consume. You want to focus on adding healthy fats like olive oil, coconut oil, butter, MCT oil, high-fat cheeses, high-fat nuts and seeds (make sure they are Keto-friendly!) and so on.

Also, if you are just starting out, it's better not to worry about counting calories until you fully reach "fat adaptation" and ketosis. Focusing on consuming more healthy fats together with cutting out the carbs will make the transition go a lot faster.

Depending on your metabolism and what you eat, getting into ketosis can take you anywhere from 24 hours to a week. In addition, becoming fully fat adapted usually takes 3-6 weeks.

So, cheating can potentially undo days of consistency and hard work. Not to mention that you are very likely to get the "keto flu" like symptoms every time you cheat, and who wants to go through that just for one cheat meal? That's right, nobody.

And, I mean… you can have bacon while on Keto, which other diet allows something like that? No cheating.

Eating too much protein

For some odd reason, people often believe Keto is a high-protein diet.

Keto is actually a high-fat, low-carb, moderate-protein diet, or to be more precise, 80% of the calorie-intake should be from fats, 15% from protein and 5% from carbs (the carbs should come from nutrient-dense, low -starch veggies).

Protein is very easy to go overboard with since it's in a lot of foods, like all kinds of meats, fish, eggs, cheese, and even in nuts. And if you consume a lot of protein, the excess protein actually turns into sugar (glucose) through the process of gluconeogenesis, which can certainly knock you out of ketosis.

So, at least for a period of time, it's recommended that you track your macros until you get an idea of what foods and how much of it you should eat. Just note that unlike protein and carbs, which contain 4 calories per gram, fats contain 9 calories per gram of fat.

Not taking electrolytes

And last but not least, electrolytes.

When some people start a Keto diet, they may experience "flu" like symptoms like fatigue, headaches, diarrhea, which often makes one believe that the Keto way of eating is not right for their bodies. But this is just a transition period until you reach ketosis.

And this is because, when we completely cut out carbs, our body produces less insulin and glycogen (carbs) stores are depleted. For every gram of glycogen, three grams of water are stored as well. That's why when people start a Keto diet, for the first few days they usually lose a couple of kilograms of water weight and feel less bloated.

While looking better is the upside, the downside is, with the flush of water, electrolytes like sodium, potassium, and magnesium are excreted as well, which causes the "flu" like symptoms.

Taking electrolytes is a very easy way that will quickly fix most of these transition "side-effects." Eating bone broth daily and adding pink Himalayan salt to your foods should do the trick, but you can also take an electrolyte supplement to make the transition even smoother.

Exercise at Home

If you go to a gym or plan to start going to a gym a private trainer would be most valuable to you. Many would rather exercise at home.

The three basic things that every person who ever stepped into the gym thought about are – weight loss, reduce belly fat and burn calories.

These fundamentals are the necessary for every fitness enthusiast.

Well accomplishing all the three above mentioned task at once may seem difficult, but it is certainly not impossible. And yes, don't even think that hitting abs thrice a week would do any good to your goals.

All you need is a sound diet strategy along with rigorous workout routine to help you build a flat midsection.

WHY AEROBIC EXERCISE TO REDUCE WEIGHT IS THE BEST WAY?

Aerobic exercise which is primarily known as cardiovascular exercise or fat burning exercise is a rhythmic motion of more than one muscle groups in the body.

The reason why aerobic exercise is also known as fat burning exercise is that of its potential to use fat over carbohydrates as a fuel to keep you moving during a workout. The reason why aerobic exercise is also known as fat burning exercise is that of its potential to use fat over carbohydrates as a fuel to keep you moving during a workout

One thing's for sure, within just a few months of aerobic training, you will see your body fat drop down at a good rate. You will look good and feel energetic.

Several studies have shown a wide range of benefits of aerobic exercise concerned with protection from heart and vascular diseases.

• One way by which aerobic exercise prevents accumulation fat is by reducing the blood pressure and making the blood vessels a little stiff which also averts clogging of blood vessels.

• Moreover, prolonged exposure to aerobic training also increases the volume of the blood pumped with each heart beat. And that's the reason why pro athletes have stroke volume twice as high as people who live a sedentary lifestyle.

• As I mentioned earlier, aerobic exercise tends to rely more on fat for the fuel, and hence, it decrease the production of lactic acid which enables a person to keep going without much fatigue. In fact, your body needs an excess amount of oxygen to burn fat, high density compared to carbs. And the finest way to up the oxygen intake and burn fat simultaneously is by performing aerobic exercises regularly.

The other known benefits of aerobic exercise include reduction of mental health problems like anxiety, depression and stress. Aerobic exercise provides you with much-needed energy and stamina and thereby boosts up your mood. Moreover, a study showed that walking three to five days per week for as little 30 minutes per workout reduced scores on a depression questionnaire by 47% after twelve weeks.

HOW YOU CAN DO AEROBICS WORKOUT AT HOME

You don't necessarily need a gym membership or some personal trainer to do aerobic exercises. There are plenty of easy aerobic exercise routines which you can do in the privacy of your place and that too with your favorite music. Sounds cool isn't it?

• One way by which aerobic exercise prevents accumulation fat is by reducing the blood pressure and making the blood vessels a little stiff which also averts clogging of blood vessels.

• Moreover, prolonged exposure to aerobic training also increases the volume of the blood pumped with each heart beat. And that's the reason why pro athletes have stroke volume twice as high as people who live a sedentary lifestyle.

• As I mentioned earlier, aerobic exercise tends to rely more on fat for the fuel, and hence, it decrease the production of lactic acid which enables a person to keep going without much fatigue. In fact, your body needs an excess amount of oxygen to burn fat, high density compared to carbs. And the finest way to up the oxygen intake and burn fat simultaneously is by performing aerobic exercises regularly.

The other known benefits of aerobic exercise include reduction of mental health problems like anxiety, depression and stress. Aerobic exercise provides you with much-needed energy and stamina and thereby boosts up your mood. Moreover, a study showed that walking three to five days per week for as little 30 minutes per workout reduced scores on a depression questionnaire by 47% after twelve weeks.

Check Your Weight Daily

Date **Weight** **Pounds to Go to Goal**

Check Your Weight Daily

Date   **Weight**   **Pounds to Go to Goal**

Check Your Weight Daily

Date   **Weight**   **Pounds to Go to Goal**

Check Your Weight Daily

Date   **Weight**   **Pounds to Go to Goal**

Check Your Weight Daily

Date   **Weight**   **Pounds to Go to Goal**

Check Your Weight Daily

Date   **Weight**   **Pounds to Go to Goal**

Vita-Guard Keto Foods

Check Your Weight Daily

Date   **Weight**   **Pounds to Go to Goal**

Check Your Weight Daily

Date   **Weight**   **Pounds to Go to Goal**

____

____

____

____

____

____

____

____

____

____

____

Food Journal

Date   **Foods Consumed**

____

____

____

____

____

____

____

____

____

____

____

____

Food Journal

Date   **Foods Consumed**

____

____

____

____

____

____

____

____

____

____

____

Food Journal

Date   **Foods Consumed**

Food Journal

Date   **Foods Consumed**

____

____

____

____

____

____

____

____

____

____

____

____

Food Journal

Date   **Foods Consumed**

Food Journal

Date   **Foods Consumed**

____

____

____

____

____

____

____

____

____

____

____

____

Food Journal

Date   **Foods Consumed**

____

____

____

____

____

____

____

____

____

____

____

____

Food Journal

Date   **Foods Consumed**

Food Journal

Date   **Foods Consumed**

Other Vita-Guard Products

Vita-Guard Arthritis Formula

Vita-Guard Wellness Formula

Vita-Guard Horny Goat Weed

Vita-Guard Vitamins & Minerals

Website: www.Vita-Guard.com

Email: vitaguard1912@gmail.com

Vita-Guard Products

91 E. Main Street

Inman, SC 29349

Visit one of our FREE training meetings

9 781796 322576